CLINICAL ACTIVITIES TO A[C]

THERAPEUTIC MODALITIES

THE ART AND SCIENCE

KENNETH L. KNIGHT
DAVID O. DRAPER

Kenneth L. Knight, PhD, ATC, FACSM
Jesse Knight Professor of Exercise Sciences
Department of Exercise Sciences
College of Health and Human Performance
Brigham Young University
Provo, Utah

David O. Draper, EdD, ATC, LAT
Professor of Exercise Sciences
Department of Exercise Sciences
College of Health and Human Performance
Brigham Young University
Provo, Utah

Wolters Kluwer | Lippincott Williams & Wilkins
Health
Philadelphia · Baltimore · New York · London
Buenos Aires · Hong Kong · Sydney · Tokyo

Acquisitions Editor: Emily Lupash
Managing Editor: Meredith Brittain
Marketing Manager: Christen Murphy
Production Editor: Julie Montalbano
Designer: Terry Mallon
Photographer: Mark A. Philbrick
Compositor: Maryland Composition, Inc.

9 8 7 6 5 4 3 2 1

Disclaimer

Care has been taken to confirm the accuracy of the information present and to describe generally accepted practices. However, the authors, editors, and publisher are not responsible for errors or omissions or for any consequences from application of the information in this book and make no warranty, expressed or implied, with respect to the currency, completeness, or accuracy of the contents of the publication. Application of this information in a particular situation remains the professional responsibility of the practitioner; the clinical treatments described and recommended may not be considered absolute and universal recommendations.

The authors, editors, and publisher have exerted every effort to ensure that drug selection and dosage set forth in this text are in accordance with the current recommendations and practice at the time of publication. However, in view of ongoing research, changes in government regulations, and the constant flow of information relating to drug therapy and drug reactions, the reader is urged to check the package insert for each drug for any change in indications and dosage and for added warnings and precautions. This is particularly important when the recommended agent is a new or infrequently employed drug.

Some drugs and medical devices presented in this publication have Food and Drug Administration (FDA) clearance for limited use in restricted research settings. It is the responsibility of the health care provider to ascertain the FDA status of each drug or device planned for use in their clinical practice.

To purchase additional copies of this book, call our customer service department at (800) 638-3030 or fax orders to (301) 223-2320. International customers should call (301) 223-2300.

Visit Lippincott Williams & Wilkins on the Internet: http://www.lww.com. Lippincott Williams & Wilkins customer service representatives are available from 8:30 am to 6:00 pm, EST.

Introduction: How to Use This Workbook

Clinical Activities to Accompany Therapeutic Modalities: The Art and Science is divided into two major sections:

- Discovery Activities
- Application Proficiency Activities

There are 18 discovery activities designed to help students discover through experience the concepts taught in the text. The 16 application proficiency activities help students develop proficiency in applying various therapeutic modalities with the 5-step application process.

Discovery Activities

Each discovery activity begins with a scenario that presents the clinical context of the activity. The purpose statement is then explained. Next, there is a list of materials needed to complete the activity, which will assist the course instructor by enabling him/her to acquire the items needed in advance for the lab. This is followed by a clearly outlined set of directions. When the activity is finished, a set of open-ended questions follow to test critical thinking skills. Finally, charts or graphs that are necessary to complete the activity are included at the end.

Application Proficiency Activities

The activities of this unit help you to develop proficiency in applying various therapeutic modalities with the 5-step application process. For each modality, study the material in the text relating to the modality, then practice applying the modality until you feel you can do so without consulting your book or notes. Then apply the modality to a classmate, who will check (or circle the number of) the tasks as you perform them correctly and in a reasonably correct order. After you finish, discuss your performance with the classmate, with specific emphasis on those tasks you missed or performed incorrectly. Repeat a second time on another day.

Contents

Application Proficiency Activities

Discovery Activities

Records Search

Textbook Reference: Part I, Chapter 3

Name: _____

Date: _____

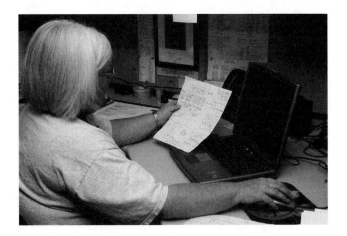

CONTEXT

Record keeping is essential and complex. To keep proper records, you must become familiar with the record-keeping system and individual records used by your specific job site. Numerous types of records are discussed in Chapter 3. This activity is designed to help you make the information in Chapter 3 operational by discovering the specific system and records of your clinical education sites.

PURPOSE

Your objective is to collect a copy of each record in each of the clinical education sites to which you may be assigned and classify the records according to the criteria presented in Chapter 3 of your text.

MATERIALS

None

DIRECTIONS

1. Visit each clinical site assigned by your instructor. At each:
   a. Introduce yourself to the person in charge and tell them you are completing an activity for your Therapeutic Modalities class. Ask if you can have copies of each of the records used by that clinic.
   b. Determine the purpose of each record. Construct a table for the purpose of the report with rows for each record; organizing by clinic or type of record will help you visualize the project.
   c. Write a brief report concerning your experience and include the table.

Comparing Various Ways of Providing Compression When Using RICES

Texbook Reference: Part II, Chapters 5–6

Name: _____

Date: _____

CONTEXT

We all know the importance of compression during immediate care of acute injury. Typically this involves using an elastic wrap to secure an ice bag directly on the skin. Unfortunately some people are of the opinion that an ice bag applied directly to the skin will damage the tissue. They suggest that a small towel or one layer of the elastic wrap first be applied to the area before the ice bag is applied. We don't believe this will provide enough of the tissue cooling needed for acute injuries. Since students may be exposed to both of these techniques, how can they understand which technique is preferred? Which one provides the greatest cooling or numbing of the area?

PURPOSE

Your objective is to compare the sensation of cold, numbing, and skin temperature change during RICES, using two different compression techniques.

MATERIALS

Crushed ice packs
Elastic wraps (4" double length preferred)
Small towel or washcloth
Flexible skin temperature measuring device
Numerical rating scale (0–10)
Temperature recording scale

DIRECTIONS

1. Have your partner sit on a table with an ankle exposed.
2. Using the numerical rating scale, have your partner rate his/her sensation at normal (10).
3. Attach the skin temperature thermometer to the skin near the lateral malleolus and tape in place. (Leave the tip exposed, do not cover with tape.)

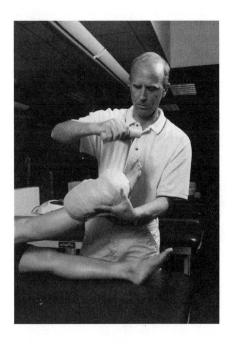

4. Record a baseline skin temperature.
5. Apply a crushed ice pack to the ankle.
6. Apply an elastic wrap to the area, overlapping half each time and pulling with moderate tension.
7. Leave the wrap on for 30 minutes.
8. Ask your partner to rate his/her sensation of cold/numbness at 5, 10, 15, 20, 25, and 30 minutes.
9. Record skin temperature at 5, 10, 15, 20, 25, and 30 minutes.
10. Remove the ice and wrap.
11. Repeat steps 1–10 on the opposite ankle; however, place one layer of the small towel or washcloth over the thermometer before applying the elastic wrap.
12. Clean up the area.
13. Compare the findings on the charts.

Questions

1. What did you learn from this experience?

   _____

   _____

   _____

2. Which modality provided the most cold/numbing?

_____

_____

_____

3. What are the advantages of each modality?

_____

_____

_____

4. What are the weaknesses of each modality?

_____

_____

_____

5. How can you use this information for treating future patients?

_____

_____

_____

Numbing Sensory Rating Scale										
0	1	2	3	4	5	6	7	8	9	10
no sensation		quite numb			moderately numb		mildly numb			normal sensation

Directions: For each of the times below, determine the number that best describes your level of sensation/numbing and write it in the appropriate blank.

Baseline temp.: _____ 5 min: _____ 10 min: _____ 15 min: _____ 20 min: _____ 25 min: _____ 30 min: _____

Comparing Elastic Wraps and Plastic Wraps on a Spool for Providing Compression

Textbook Reference: Part II, Chapters 5–6

Name: _____

Date: _____

CONTEXT

We all know the importance of compression during immediate care of acute injury. Typically this involves using an elastic wrap to secure an ice bag directly on the skin. Another popular method of applying ice packs is with plastic wraps that come on a spool. Though convenient for holding ice in place, research has shown that these plastic wraps don't provide enough compression needed for acute injuries. Since students will be exposed to both of these techniques, how can they understand which technique is preferred? Which one provides the greatest cooling or numbing of the area?

PURPOSE

Your objective is to compare the sensation of cold, numbing, and skin temperature change during RICES, using different compression techniques.

MATERIALS

Crushed ice packs
Elastic wraps (4" double length preferred)
Plastic wrap on a spool
Flexible skin temperature measuring device
Numerical rating scale (0–10)
Temperature recording scale

DIRECTIONS

1. Have your partner sit on a table with an ankle exposed.
2. Using the numerical rating scale, have your partner rate his/her sensation at normal (10).
3. Attach the skin temperature thermometer to the skin near the lateral malleolus and tape in place. (Leave the tip exposed, do not cover with tape.)
4. Record a baseline skin temperature.
5. Apply a crushed ice pack to the ankle.

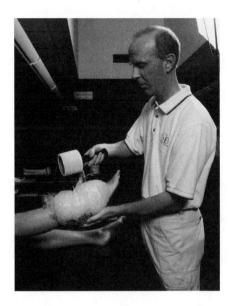

6. Apply an elastic wrap to the area, overlapping half each time and pulling with moderate tension.
7. Keep the wrap on for 30 minutes.
8. Ask your partner to rate his/her sensation of cold/numbness at 5, 10, 15, 20, 25, and 30 minutes.
9. Record skin temperature at 5, 10, 15, 20, 25, and 30 minutes.
10. Remove the ice and wrap.
11. Repeat steps 1–10 on the opposite ankle; however, use the plastic wrap on a spool instead of the elastic wrap.
12. Clean up the area.
13. Compare the findings on the charts.

Questions

1. What did you learn from this experience?

   _____

   _____

   _____

2. Which modality provided the most cold/numbing?

   _____

   _____

   _____

3. What are the advantages of each modality?

_____

_____

_____

4. What are the weaknesses of each modality?

_____

_____

_____

5. How can you use this information for treating future patients?

_____

_____

_____

Numbing Sensory Rating Scale										
0	1	2	3	4	5	6	7	8	9	10
no sensation		quite numb			moderately numb		mildly numb			normal sensation

Directions: For each of the times below, determine the number that best describes your level of sensation/numbing and write it in the appropriate blank.

Baseline temp.: _____   5 min: _____   10 min: _____   15 min: _____   20 min: _____   25 min: _____   30 min: _____

Electrical Stimulation Electrode Application Parameters

Textbook Reference: Part IV, Chapters 9–10

Name: _____

Date: _____

CONTEXT

Many parameters affect electrical stimulation, and the way that electrodes are applied influences those parameters.

PURPOSE

Your objective is to compare the sensation of, and muscular contraction during, various neuromuscular electrical application stimulation parameters.

MATERIALS

An electrical neuromuscular stimulation unit
A pair of bipolar electrodes

DIRECTIONS

1. Using bipolar electrodes, firmly attach one electrode on one forearm. Lay the second electrode on a table with the active side up.
2. Place the palm of your hand firmly on the second electrode.
3. Set up
   a. Wave form: bipolar
   b. Frequency: 2–3 cps
4. Increase the output intensity until you feel a moderate current.
5. Explore the following. Return to the above conditions after each activity so that each activity begins the same way.
   a. Current density—slide your hand from the second electrode until only the tip of your index finger is in contact with the electrode. How did the current sensation change at the forearm and at the finger? Why? Would this still be considered a bipolar application?

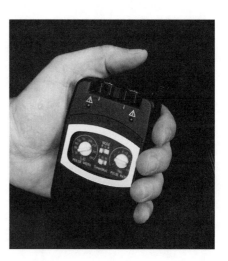

   b. Effect of pulse rate—gradually increase the pulse rate until you invoke a tetanic contraction, then decrease to 2–3 cps. At what pulse rate did you feel the strongest contraction?
   c. Electrode application—(you must have non-adhesive electrodes for this activity). Place your second forearm on the table.
      i) Lay the second electrode on the forearm. Note the current intensity and strength of contraction.
      ii) Firmly attach the second electrode to the forearm with an elastic belt or elastic wrap. Note the current intensity and strength of contraction.
      iii) Place a moistened paper towel or sponge on the forearm and then firmly attach the second electrode to the forearm with an elastic belt or elastic wrap. Note the current intensity and strength of contraction.
      iv) How did the current intensity and strength of contraction change from Step 5.c.(i) to 5.c.(iii)? What part of Ohm's law changed as you progressed through these steps? Why is it important to firmly attach electrodes?

Finding Optimal Electrode Placement Sites (Motor Points)

Textbook Reference: Part IV, Chapters 9–10

Name: _____

Date: _____

CONTEXT

It is often difficult to find the best place to apply an electrode. Many clinicians will place one on the muscle belly and another distal or proximal to it, only to find very little current flowing through the area. He/she then has to move the electrode, turn up the intensity and try again. There is a faster, more effective way to find motor points.

PURPOSE

This lab will assist you in finding the best place to apply electrodes for optimal current flow.

MATERIALS

E-stim unit (or TENS unit)
Alcohol swabs
Electrodes

DIRECTIONS

1. Using the alcohol swab, clean the area on your partner where you want to apply the two electrodes.
2. Apply one electrode on your partner's muscle belly. This is typically where one motor point is.
3. Apply the other electrode to the back of your hand or arm.
4. Apply a liberal amount of electrode or ultrasound gel to your second and third fingers.
5. Using your second and third fingers, touch the muscle attachment of the muscles you want to stimulate. (For example, if you want to cause wrist extension, the electrode would be on the wrist extensor's muscle belly and you would touch this muscle's attachment just distal to the lateral epicondyle.)
6. Slowly turn up the intensity until you see the muscle twitch.
7. Slowly move your fingers around searching for the strongest sensation or contraction.

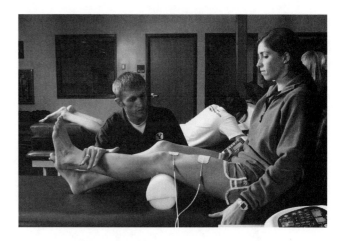

8. The site of the strongest sensation or contraction is the second motor point.
9. Turn the intensity back to zero.
10. Attach the second electrode to this spot and slowly turn up the intensity.

Questions

1. What did you learn from this experience?

_____

_____

_____

2. What did you have to do to complete the circuit?

_____

_____

_____

Comparing Old and New Reusable Electrodes

Textbook Reference: Part IV, Chapters 9–10

Name: _____

Date: _____

CONTEXT

Many clinicians get into the habit of using self-adhering reusable electrodes well beyond their shelf life. After 7 to 10 uses, these not only lose their adhesive properties but they might also lose the ability to conduct an adequate current to the patient.

PURPOSE

This lab will help you to realize the importance of using fairly new, properly maintained electrodes.

MATERIALS

E-stim unit
Alcohol swabs
Reusable self-adhering electrodes (same size):
- new
- used 10 or more times

Chart with following listed:
- μamps to sensation
- μamps to muscle twitch
- μamps to muscle contraction

DIRECTIONS

1. Using the alcohol swab, clean an area on your partner where a muscle stimulation unit or TENS unit might produce a muscle contraction.
2. Apply two new electrodes of the same size to the area. Attach the electrodes to the leads and the leads to the unit.
3. Adjust the pulse frequency to 80–100 pps.
4. Slowly adjust the intensity (μamps) until your partner first notices the current sensation. Write the μamps on your chart by sensation.
5. Slowly adjust the intensity (μamps) until you and your partner first notice a muscle twitch. Write the μamps on your chart by muscle twitch.

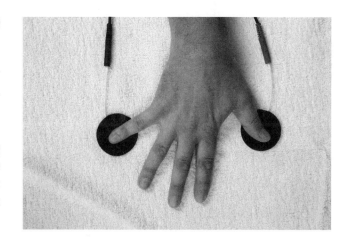

6. Slowly adjust the intensity (μamps) until you and your partner first notice a full muscle contraction. Write the μamps on your chart by muscle contraction.
7. Turn the intensity to zero and the unit off. Replace the electrodes with the used electrodes and repeat steps 3–6.
8. Turn the intensity to zero and the unit off.
9. Clean off the treatment area and put the unit away.

Questions

1. What did you learn from this experience?

_____

_____

_____

2. How can you apply what you have just learned in your future setting?

_____

_____

_____

Comparing Single-Use with Reusable Electrodes

Textbook Reference: Part IV, Chapters 9–10

Name: _____

Date: _____

CONTEXT

In many athletic training settings, self-adhering reusable electrodes are not only used beyond their normal shelf-life, but one pair may be used on several patients. This can produce cross-contamination and spread of germs. A few companies are now producing single-use electrodes that are discarded after one use. How do these single-use electrodes compare to the traditional self-adhering electrodes that have been used several times?

PURPOSE

The purpose of this lab is to see if single-use electrodes produce as strong of a current as a well-used reusable self-adhering electrode.

MATERIALS

E-stim unit
Alcohol swabs
Reusable self-adhering electrodes used 10 or more times
Single-use, self-adhering electrodes
Chart with following listed:
- μamps to sensation
- μamps to muscle twitch
- μamps to muscle contraction

DIRECTIONS

1. Using the alcohol swab, clean an area on your partner where a muscle stimulation unit or TENS unit might produce a muscle contraction.
2. Apply two single-use electrodes of the same size to the area. Attach the electrodes to the leads and the leads to the unit.
3. Adjust the pulse frequency to 80–100 pps.
4. Slowly adjust the intensity (μamps) until your partner first notices the current sensation. Write the μamps on your chart by sensation.

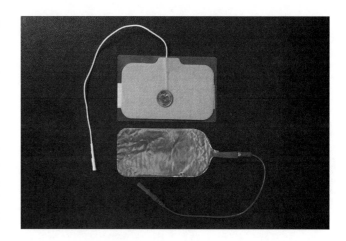

5. Slowly adjust the intensity (μamps) until you and your partner first notice a muscle twitch. Write the μamps on your chart by muscle twitch.
6. Slowly adjust the intensity (μamps) until you and your partner first notice a full muscle contraction. Write the μamps on your chart by muscle contraction.
7. Turn the intensity to zero and the unit off. Replace the electrodes with the used electrodes and repeat steps 3–6. (Note: If the used electrodes are not the same size as the new ones, trim them to the same size before attaching to your partner.)
8. Turn the intensity to zero and the unit off.
9. Clean off the treatment area and put the unit away.

Questions

1. What did you learn from this experience?

   _____

   _____

   _____

2. How can you apply what you have just learned in your future setting?

   _____

   _____

Iontophoresis to Reduce Scar Tissue/Adhesions

ACTIVITY

8

Textbook Reference: Part IV, Chapters 9–10

Name: _____

Date: _____

CONTEXT

Acetic acid is used with iontophoresis to soften scar tissue. This might be difficult to demonstrate on a student without scar tissue. One possible way might be by using a substance very close to acetic acid—vinegar.

PURPOSE

The objective of this lab is to demonstrate the procedure used to deliver vinegar via iontophoresis and determine whether this will soften calluses.

MATERIALS

Iontophoresor
Electrodes
Alcohol swab
Pen
Vinegar
Syringe
Cotton swab

DIRECTIONS

1. With a partner, take a cotton swab and find an area on the palms of the hands or bottom of the feet where there are some calluses.
    a. Probe this area with the cotton swab to determine the hardness of a callus.
    b. Clean this area with an alcohol swab.
2. Use the syringe to extract 1 ml of vinegar from a bottle of vinegar.
    a. Apply vinegar to the delivery electrode.
    b. Attach delivery electrode to the skin over and around the callus.
    c. Attach dispersive electrode about 6" away on a fleshy area.
    d. Attach electrode clips on electrodes and unit.
3. Increase power to patient tolerance.

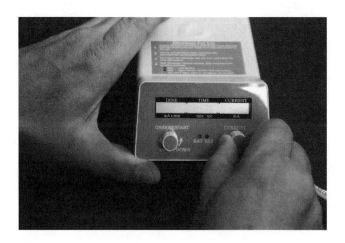

4. Deliver the treatment dose (10–20 min depending on intensity).
5. When the machine shuts off:
    a. Quickly remove drug delivery electrode.
    b. Probe the callus with the cotton swab using the same amount of pressure as you did before.
    c. Clean up the entire area and put the unit away.

Questions

1. Did the callus get any softer? (Note: This may take several treatments.)

    _____

    _____

    _____

2. Did the treatment area feel any softer to your partner?

    _____

    _____

    _____

3. How could you use this technique to help your patients?

    _____

    _____

    _____

Iontophoresis to Produce Numbness

Textbook Reference: Part IV, Chapters 9–10

Name: _____

Date: _____

CONTEXT

Pain relief is a very difficult thing to measure. One possible way is to see how much of an area can be numbed.

PURPOSE

The objective of this lab is to see if iontophoresis with lidocaine can produce numbness on a muscle.

MATERIALS

Iontophoresor
Electrodes
Alcohol swab
Pen
Lidocaine
Syringe
Paperclip
Visual analog or numerical scale

DIRECTIONS

1. Using a partner, take an alcohol swab and clean an area of the wrist extensors on the muscles of the forearm about 2" distal to the lateral epicondyle.
2. Open an end of the paperclip.
   a. Provide firm pressure on the muscles of the forearm with the paperclip, and mark this spot with a pen.
   b. Have your partner rate how much pain he/she experienced using the VAS or numerical scale.
3. Use the syringe to extract 1 ml of lidocaine from the bottle.
   a. Apply lidocaine to the delivery electrode.
   b. Attach delivery electrode to the skin when the pen mark is.
   c. Attach dispersive electrode about 6" away on the deltoid area.

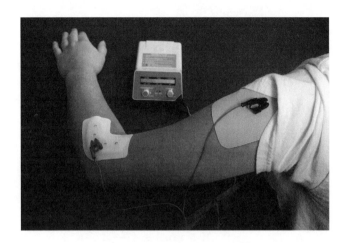

   d. Attach electrode clips on electrodes and unit (positive delivery method).
4. Increase power to patient tolerance.
5. Deliver the treatment dose (10–20 min depending on intensity).
6. When the machine shuts off:
   a. Quickly remove drug delivery electrode.
   b. Apply the same amount of pressure with the paperclip as you did before.
   c. Have your partner rate how much pain they are now experiencing using the VAS or numerical scale.

Questions

1. Did the area decrease in sensation from the treatment?

   _____

   _____

   _____

2. How could you use this technique to help your patients?

   _____

   _____

   _____

Comparing Intensity and Duration of Heat Sensation Provided by Various Heat Modalities

Textbook Reference: Part V, Chapters 11–12

Name: _____

Date: _____

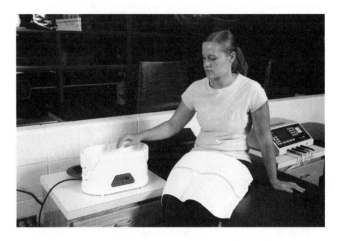

CONTEXT

There are several superficial heating modalities used in clinical and sports settings. Some are easier to use than others, but which one provides the greatest sensation of heat? Which lasts the longest?

PURPOSE

Your objective is to compare the sensation of heat provided by several superficial heating modalities.

MATERIALS

Silicate gel hot pack and container
Warm whirlpool
Paraffin bath
Numerical rating scale (0–10)

DIRECTIONS

1. Have your partner sit on a table.
2. Using the numerical rating scale, have your partner rate his/her sensation of heat at normal (0).
3. Apply a standard silicate gel hot pack in its terry cloth cover to the back of the hand for 10 minutes. Apply another layer of toweling between the skin and pack if the area gets too hot.
4. Ask your partner to rate his/her sensation of heat at 5, 10, 15, and 20 minutes.
5. Dip your partners hand in a paraffin bath 7–10 times/layers.
6. Carefully place the wax-coated hand in a plastic bag and cover with a towel.
7. Ask your partner to rate his/her sensation of heat at 5 and 10 minutes.
8. Remove the wax glove after 10 minutes.

9. Have your partner continue to rate his/her sensation of heat at 15 and 20 minutes.
10. Immerse your partner's hand in a warm/hot whirlpool for 10 minutes.
11. Ask your partner to rate his/her sensation of heat at 5, 10, 15, and 20 minutes.
12. Clean up the area.
13. Compare the findings on the charts.

Questions

1. What did you learn from this experience?

   _____

   _____

   _____

2. Which modality provided the most heat?

   _____

   _____

   _____

3. Which modality provided the longest lasting heating?

   _____

   _____

   _____

4. What are the advantages of each modality?

    _____

    _____

    _____

5. What are the weaknesses of each modality?

    _____

    _____

    _____

6. How can you use this information for treating future patients?

    _____

    _____

    _____

Heat Sensory Rating Scale										
0	1	2	3	4	5	6	7	8	9	10
no heat		mild warmth			moderately warm		very warm			hot

Directions: For each of the times below, determine the number that best describes your level of sensation/heat and write it in the appropriate blank.

Baseline temp.: _____   5 min: _____   10 min: _____   15 min: _____   20 min: _____

Comparing Intensity and Duration of Heat Provided by Various Wraps, Plasters, and Patches

Textbook Reference: Part V, Chapters 11–12

Name: _____

Date: _____

CONTEXT

Several radio and television advertisements claim that menthol- or capsaicin-based products relieve pain or produce heat. We have researched several of these products and, while all produce a sensation of heat, only the ThermaCare actually produces mild heat in the muscles. Herein lies the problem: both menthol- and capsaicin-based products make the skin feel warm, but is that enough to relieve the pain?

PURPOSE

Your objective is to compare the sensation of heat provided by several wraps, plasters, and patches and determine if they have a place in allied health and sports medicine.

MATERIALS

Heat wrap (such as the ThermaCare HeatWrap discussed in Chapter 12). Note: The ThermaCare HeatWrap must be taken out of the package 30 min prior to the experiment.
Back plaster (capsaicin-based; a derivative of the hot pepper plant)
Pain or heat patch(es)
Numerical rating scale (0–10)
Pen

DIRECTIONS

1. Have your partner lie prone on a table.
2. Have your partner rate his/her sensation of heat at normal (0).
3. Apply similarly sized heat wrap, plaster, or patch to the area.
4. Ask your partner to rate his/her sensation of heat at 5, 10, 15, 20, 25, and 30 minutes.
5. Remove the product without showing it to your partner.

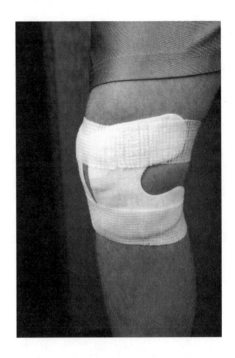

6. Repeat steps 2–5 with another product.
7. Repeat steps 2–5 with another product.
8. Clean up the area.
9. Compare the findings on the charts.

Questions

1. What did you learn from this experience?

_____

_____

_____

2. How could the placebo effect be both useful and detrimental when using these products?

_____

_____

_____

Heat Sensory Rating Scale										
0	1	2	3	4	5	6	7	8	9	10
no heat		mild warmth			moderately warm		very warm			hot

Directions: For each of the times below, determine the number that best describes your level of sensation/heat and write it in the appropriate blank.

Baseline temp.: _____   5 min: _____   10 min: _____   15 min: _____   20 min: _____   25 min: _____   30 min: _____

Comparing Intensity and Duration of Heat Provided by Various Sports Creams and a Placebo

Textbook Reference: Part V, Chapters 11–12

Name: _____

Date: _____

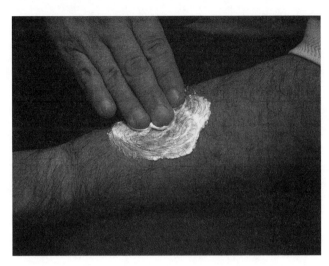

CONTEXT

Several radio and television advertisements claim that menthol- or capsaicin-based products relieve pain and/or produce heat. We have researched several of these products and, while all produce a sensation of heat, is the heat enough to relieve the pain?

PURPOSE

Your objective is to compare the sensation of heat provided by several sports creams and to see if the placebo can be detected.

MATERIALS

Two or three sports creams with menthol or capsaicin as the active ingredient.
Placebo cream (ultrasound lotion, massage lotion, etc.)
Numerical rating scale (0–10)
Pen

DIRECTIONS

1. Have your partner lie prone on a table.
2. Use the pen to trace a 6 x 6 inch area on your partner's back, calf or hamstring.
3. Have your partner rate his/her sensation of heat at normal (0).
4. Apply some of the sports cream (or placebo) to the area and gently massage this into the muscle for 2 minutes. Reapply if needed.
5. Ask your partner to rate his/her sensation of heat at 5 and 10 minutes.
6. Repeat steps 2–5 on another area.
7. When finished, repeat steps 2–5 on another area.
8. Clean up the area.
9. Compare the findings on the charts.

Questions

1. What did you learn from this experience?

   _____

   _____

   _____

2. Did you or your partner correctly identify the placebo?

   _____

   _____

   _____

3. How can you use this information for treating future patients?

   _____

   _____

   _____

Heat Sensory Rating Scale										
0	1	2	3	4	5	6	7	8	9	10
no heat		mild warmth			moderately warm		very warm			hot

Directions: For each of the times below, determine the number that best describes your level of sensation/heat and write it in the appropriate blank.

Baseline temp.: _____ 5 min: _____ 10 min: _____

Comparing Intensity and Duration of Cold Sensation Provided by Various Cold Modalities

Textbook Reference: Part V, Chapters 13–14

Name: _____

Date: _____

CONTEXT

There are several superficial cooling modalities used in the clinical and sports settings. Some are easier to use than others, but which one provides the greatest cooling or numbing of the area? Which lasts the longest?

PURPOSE

Your objective is to compare the sensation of cold and numbing provided by several superficial cooling modalities.

MATERIALS

Crushed ice pack
Cold whirlpool
Ice massage cup
Ice slush bath
Numerical rating scale (0–10)

DIRECTIONS

1. Have your partner sit on a table or stool convenient to the treatment area.
2. Using the numerical rating scale, have your partner rate his/her sensation at normal (10).
3. Apply a crushed ice pack to an extremity for 10–15 min (with or without a wrap).
4. Ask your partner to rate his/her sensation of cold/numbness at 5, 10, 15, and 20 minutes.
5. Apply the second modality for the same time period and repeat steps 2 and 4.
6. Apply the third modality for the same time period and repeat steps 2 and 4.
7. Apply the fourth modality for the same time period and repeat steps 2 and 4.
8. Clean up the area.
9. Compare the findings on the charts.

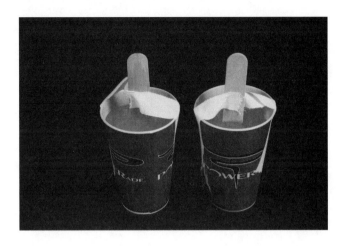

Questions

1. What did you learn from this experience?

   _____

   _____

   _____

2. Which modality provided the most cold/numbing?

   _____

   _____

   _____

3. Which modality provided the longest lasting cold/numbing?

   _____

   _____

   _____

4. What are the advantages of each modality?

   _____

   _____

   _____

5. What are the weaknesses of each modality?

_____

_____

_____

6. How can you use this information for treating future patients?

_____

_____

_____

Numbing Sensory Rating Scale

0	1	2	3	4	5	6	7	8	9	10
no sensation		quite numb			moderately numb		mildly numb			normal sensation

Directions: For each of the times below, determine the number that best describes your level of sensation/numbing and write it in the appropriate blank.

Baseline temp.: _____   5 min: _____   10 min: _____   15 min: _____   20 min: _____

ACTIVITY

14

Comparing Intensity of Cold Sensation from Ice Immersion with and without a Neoprene Toe Cap

Textbook Reference: Part V, Chapters 13–14

Name: _____

Date: _____

CONTEXT

Cryotherapy is very beneficial for numbing an area prior to exercise. Often, the ankle needs to be cooled, but the toes don't need to be. This activity will help the student understand the benefits of using a toe cap to prevent the toes from getting needlessly chilled during cryotherapy.

PURPOSE

Your objective is to compare the sensation of cold and numbing during ice immersion of one bare foot and one with the toes covered with a neoprene toe cap.

MATERIALS

Ice slush bath
Neoprene toe cap
Numerical rating scale (0–10)
Paper clip

DIRECTIONS

1. Have your partner sit in a chair or stool convenient to the treatment area.
2. Use an opened paper clip and apply it to his/her toes until he/she can feel it normally.
3. Using the numerical rating scale, have your partner rate his/her sensation.
4. Apply a neoprene toe cap snugly to one foot.
5. Immerse both ankles into ice water.
6. At 15 minutes, remove both ankles from water.
7. Carefully wipe off water and apply the paper clip on toes of immersed ankle and rate sensation.
8. Carefully wipe off water and take toe cap off.
9. Apply the paper clip on toes of immersed ankle and rate sensation.
10. Clean up the area.
11. Compare the findings on the charts.

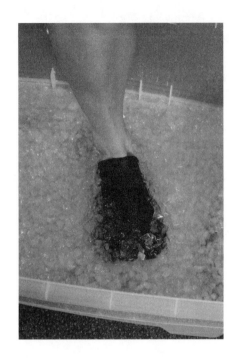

Questions

1. What did you learn from this experience?

   _____

   _____

   _____

2. What color were the toes that were exposed to the cold?

   _____

   _____

   _____

3. What color were the toes that were insulated from the cold?

   _____

   _____

   _____

4.   Are there advantages to the toe cap?

_____

_____

_____

Numbing Sensory Rating Scale										
0	1	2	3	4	5	6	7	8	9	10
no sensation		quite numb			moderately numb			mildly numb		normal sensation

Directions: Determine the number that best describes your level of sensation/ numbing and write it in the appropriate blank.

Baseline temp.: _____   15 min: _____

Comparing Intensity and Duration of Heat Provided by Ultrasound via Various Coupling Mediums

Textbook Reference: Part V, Chapter 15

Name: _____

Date: _____

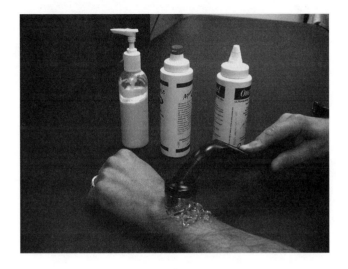

CONTEXT

From several research studies, we know that ultrasound can produce deep heat in muscles. Sometimes the patient can't feel much heat and might rely more on sports cream because he/she thinks the area will be appropriately warmed. Through laboratory research, we have found that a mixture of one part Flex-all with three parts ultrasound gel is an adequate ultrasound couplant. Will this mixture also make the patient feel warm due to the menthol in the cream?

PURPOSE

Your objective is to see if a mixture of one part menthol-based sports cream and three parts ultrasound gel produces more or less heat sensation than pure ultrasound gel during and after an ultrasound treatment.

MATERIALS

Ultrasound unit
Ultrasound gel
Mixture of menthol-based sports cream and ultrasound gel (1:3)
Numerical rating scale (0–10)
Pen

DIRECTIONS

1. Have your partner lie prone on a table.
2. Using the pen, trace an area twice the size of the ultrasound head on your partner's calf (or some other area that he/she cannot see).
3. Apply a generous amount of ultrasound gel to the treatment site.
4. Touch the soundhead to the skin.
5. Have your partner rate his/her sensation of heat at normal (0).
6. While slowly moving the soundhead back and forth in the tracing, apply the following parameters:
   a. Continuous
   b. 1MHz
   c. 1.2–1.7W/cm2
   d. 10–12 minutes (if partner tolerates)
7. Ask your partner to rate his/her sensation of heat at 5, 10, 15, and 20 minutes.
8. Repeat steps 3–6 with the sports cream/ultrasound gel mixture.
9. Clean up the area and put away the device.
10. Compare the findings on the charts.

Questions

1. What did you learn from this experience?

   _____

   _____

   _____

2. How could the placebo effect be both useful and detrimental when using a sports cream/gel mixture?

   _____

   _____

   _____

Heat Sensory Rating Scale										
0	1	2	3	4	5	6	7	8	9	10
no heat		mild warmth			moderately warm		very warm			hot

Directions: For each of the times below, determine the number that best describes your level of sensation/heat and write it in the appropriate blank.

Baseline temp.: _____ 5 min: _____ 10 min: _____ 15 min: _____ 20 min: _____

Comparing Intensity of Heat Sensation Provided by Ultrasound at 1MHz and 3MHz

Textbook Reference: Part V, Chapter 15

Name: _____

Date: _____

CONTEXT

From several research studies, we know that 3MHz ultrasound heats 3 times faster than 1MHz ultrasound. 3MHz ultrasound is also absorbed more superficially, which can be problematic if overheating takes place.

PURPOSE

Your objective is to see if your partner can feel the difference between a 1MHz and 3MHz ultrasound treatment via heat sensation.

MATERIALS

Ultrasound unit
Ultrasound gel
Numerical rating scale (0–10)
Pen

DIRECTIONS

1. Have your partner lie prone on a table.
2. Using the pen, trace an area twice the size of the ultrasound head on your partner's calf (or some other area that he/she cannot see).
3. Apply a generous amount of ultrasound gel to the treatment site.
4. Touch the soundhead to the skin.
5. Have your partner rate his/her sensation of heat.
6. While slowly moving the soundhead back and forth in the tracing, apply the following parameters:
   a. Continuous
   b. 1MHz
   c. 1W/cm^2
   d. 8–10 min (if partner tolerates). Turn off at 10 minutes.

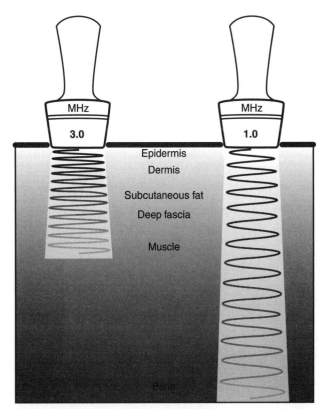

(Adapted with permission from Castel, D. International Academy of Physio Therapeutics. Clip Art.)

7. Ask your partner to rate his/her sensation of heat at 5 and 10 minutes.
8. Repeat steps 3–7 with the ultrasound machine at 3MHz at the following parameters:
   a. Continuous
   b. 1W/cm^2
   c. 8–10 min (if partner tolerates). Turn off at 10 minutes.
9. Clean up the area and put the device away.
10. Compare the findings on the charts.

Questions

1. What did you learn from this experience?

_____

_____

_____

2. How could this information affect future treatments?

_____

_____

_____

Heat Sensory Rating Scale										
0	1	2	3	4	5	6	7	8	9	10
no heat		mild warmth			moderately warm		very warm			hot

Directions: For each of the times below, determine the number that best describes your level of sensation/heat and write it in the appropriate blank.

Baseline temp.: _____ 5 min: _____ 10 min: _____

Comparing So-Called Coupling Mediums in Their Ability to Conduct Ultrasound

Textbook Reference: Part V, Chapter 15

Name: _____

Date: _____

CONTEXT

Ultrasound cannot be transmitted through the air. In order for ultrasound to be generated to the tissues, a thin layer of couplant must be placed between the skin and the soundhead. Some make the mistake in assuming that any gel-like substance can be used as a couplant.

PURPOSE

Your objective is to test various gels, creams, and lotions in a tape tube to see if they will produce ultrasound bubbles in water on top of the gel. If the water bubbles, the gel is conducting the soundwave. If few or no bubbles are produced, the sound is being blocked by the gel.

MATERIALS

Ultrasound unit
Ultrasound gel
Other gels, creams, petroleum jelly, etc.
Tape
Small glass of water
Tongue depressor

DIRECTIONS

1. Use the tape, and encircle the ultrasound head with the tape, leaving at least one-half inch exposed at the top.
2. Apply about one-quarter inch of ultrasound gel to the top of the soundhead with the tongue depressor.
3. Fill the rest of the tape tube with water.

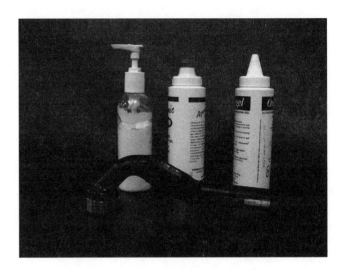

4. Set the unit on continuous and slowly turn up the intensity and record what happens? Does the ultrasound produce bubbles? Change the frequency from 1MHz to 3MHz. What change is noticed in the bubble format?
5. Turn the intensity to 0 and clean off the soundhead.
6. Apply another gel or lotion and repeat steps 3, 4, and 5.
7. Apply another gel or lotion and repeat steps 3, 4, and 5.
8. Apply petroleum jelly and repeat steps 3, 4, and 5. **Caution**: Be careful not to overheat the soundhead during this step.

Questions

1. What did you learn from this experience?

_____

_____

_____

A C T I V I T Y

18

What Healed the Lesion: The Ultrasound, the Antibiotic Ointment, or a Combination of Both?

Textbook Reference: Part V, Chapter 15

Name: _____

Date: _____

CONTEXT

A research study was published about a decade ago where an antibiotic cream was purportedly driven into the tissues via an ultrasound device. The researchers believed that the ultrasound opened up pathways in the tissues for delivery of the antibiotic drug, thus speeding up the healing at the wound site. If this were true, you should be able to make a tape tube and see if the antibiotic cream impeded or enhanced the ultrasound.

PURPOSE

Your objective is to test Bacitracin in a tape tube to see if it will produce ultrasound bubbles in water on top of it. If the water bubbles, the ointment is conducting the soundwave. If few or no bubbles are produced, the sound is being blocked by the Bacitracin.

MATERIALS

Ultrasound unit
Ultrasound gel
Bacitracin
Tape
Small glass of water
Tongue depressor

DIRECTIONS

1. Use the tape, and encircle the ultrasound head with the tape, leaving at least one-half inch exposed at the top.
2. Apply about one-quarter inch of ultrasound gel to the top of the soundhead with the tongue depressor.
3. Fill the rest of the tape tube with water.
4. Set the unit on continuous and slowly turn up the intensity and record what happens. Does the ultrasound produce bubbles? Change the frequency from

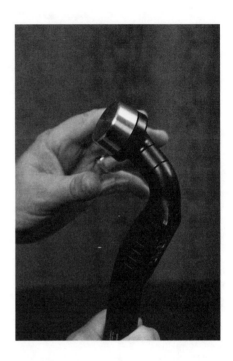

1MHz to 3MHz. What change is noticed in the bubble format?
5. Turn the intensity to 0 and clean off the soundhead.
6. Apply Bacitracin and repeat steps 3, 4, and 5. **Caution:** Be careful not to overheat the soundhead during this step.

Questions

1. What did you learn from this experience?

   _____

   _____

   _____

2. Did the original researchers make a mistake in their findings?

   _____

   _____

   _____

3. How could this impact your practice?

_____

_____

_____

Application Proficiency Activities

RICES

Textbook Reference: Part II, Chapter 5

Name: _____

	Application #	1	2

STEP 1. FOUNDATION

A. Explain RICES and basic operation — 1 2
B. Explain RICES's:
  1. Effects — 1 2
  2. Advantages — 1 2
  3. Disadvantages — 1 2
  4. Indications — 1 2
  5. Contraindications — 1 2
  6. Precautions — 1 2

STEP 2. PREAPPLICATION TASKS

A. Ensure RICES is the proper modality
  1. Reevaluate injury — 1 2
  2. Review previous application — 1 2
  3. Establish goals — 1 2
  4. Match goals to modality — 1 2
  5. Check contraindications — 1 2
B. Prepare patient psychologically
  1. Explain purpose and expected outcomes — 1 2
  2. Give brief physiology if interested — 1 2
  3. Tell what to expect, what to feel — 1 2
  4. Demonstrate on self if patient is apprehensive — 1 2
  5. Warn about precautions — 1 2
C. Prepare patient physically
  1. Remove clothing, bandages as necessary — 1 2
  2. Position patient; comfortable yet accessible — 1 2
D. Prepare equipment/supplies
  1. Set-up equipment/get supplies — 1 2
  2. Check equipment operation — 1 2
  3. Safety check — 1 2

STEP 3. APPLICATION PARAMETERS

A. Procedures
    1. Begin application   1   2
    2. Make adjustments   1   2
    3. Check patient response   1   2
B. Dosage   1   2
C. Length of application   1   2
D. Frequency of application   1   2
E. Duration of therapy   1   2

STEP 4. POSTAPPLICATION TASKS

A. Remove/replace equipment   1   2
B. Clean up patient and area   1   2
C. Instructions to patient:
    1. Schedule next treatment   1   2
    2. Level of activity   1   2
    3. Self-treatment prior to next formal treatment   1   2
    4. Physiological responses following treatment   1   2
D. Record treatment & unique responses   1   2

STEP 5. MAINTENANCE

A. Clean equipment regularly   1   2
B. Routine maintenance   1   2
C. Simple repairs   1   2

Date: _____ _____

Number correct: _____ _____

Name of Subject/Tester: _____

TENS—Pain

Textbook Reference: Part IV, Chapter 10

Name: _____

	Application #	1	2

STEP 1. FOUNDATION

A. Explain TENS and basic operation | | 1 | 2
B. Explain the NMES's:

		1	2
1.	Effects	1	2
2.	Advantages	1	2
3.	Disadvantages	1	2
4.	Indications	1	2
5.	Contraindications	1	2
6.	Precautions	1	2

STEP 2. PREAPPLICATION TASKS

A. Ensure TENS is the proper therapy

		1	2
1.	Reevaluate and review injury	1	2
2.	Review previous application	1	2
3.	Match goals to modality	1	2
4.	Select or review electrical current	1	2
5.	Check contraindications	1	2

B. Prepare patient psychologically

		1	2
1.	Explain procedure and expected outcomes	1	2
2.	Give brief physiology if interested	1	2
3.	Tell what to expect, what to feel	1	2
4.	Demonstrate on self if patient is apprehensive	1	2
5.	Warn about precautions	1	2

C. Prepare patient physically

		1	2
1.	Remove clothing, tape, as necessary	1	2
2.	Position patient; comfortable yet accessible	1	2

D. Prepare equipment/supplies

		1	2
1.	Set-up equipment/get supplies	1	2
2.	Prepare electrodes	1	2
3.	Check equipment operation	1	2
4.	Safety check	1	2

STEP 3. APPLICATION PARAMETERS

A. Procedures
    1. Set pulse rate (<10 pps for chronic pain)   1   2
    2. Set duty cycle and timer   1   2
    3. Adjust surge controls as necessary   1   2
    4. Inform patient of start/request feedback   1   2
    5. Increase until response, adjust as needed   1   2
    6. If motor point, move electrode as needed   1   2
    7. Troubleshoot discomfort   1   2
    8. Increase resistance as patient is able   1   2
B. Dosage   1   2
C. Length of application   1   2
D. Frequency of application   1   2
E. Duration of therapy   1   2

STEP 4. POSTAPPLICATION TASKS

A. Remove/replace equipment   1   2
B. Clean patient and area
C. Instructions to patient: 1   2
    1. Schedule next treatment   1   2
    2. Level of activity   1   2
    3. Self-treatment prior to next formal treatment   1   2
    4. Physiological responses following treatment   1   2
D. Record treatment and unique responses   1   2
E. Return generator cart   1   2

STEP 5. MAINTENANCE

A. Check the fuse in back of unit if not working   1   2
B. Clean equipment regularly
    1. Wash sponges or carbon-rubber electrodes   1   2
    2. Do not wash self-adhering electrodes   1   2
C. Routine maintenance
    1. Ensure wire firmly attached to electrode post   1   2
    2. Check current, assess need for new electrode   1   2

Date: _____ _____

Number correct: _____ _____

Name of Subject/Tester: _____

NMES—Tetanic Contraction

Textbook Reference: Part IV, Chapter 10

Name: _____

	Application #	1	2

STEP 1. FOUNDATION

A. Explain NMES and basic operation   1   2

B. Explain NMES's:

		1	2
1.	Effects	1	2
2.	Advantages	1	2
3.	Disadvantages	1	2
4.	Indications	1	2
5.	Contraindications	1	2
6.	Precautions	1	2

STEP 2. PREAPPLICATION TASKS

A. Ensure NMES is the proper therapy

		1	2
1.	Reevaluate and review injury	1	2
2.	Review previous application	1	2
3.	Match goals to modality	1	2
4.	Select or review electrical current	1	2
5.	Check contraindications	1	2

B. Prepare patient psychologically

		1	2
1.	Explain procedure and expected outcomes	1	2
2.	Give brief physiology if interested	1	2
3.	Tell what to expect, what to feel	1	2
4.	Demonstrate on self if patient is apprehensive	1	2
5.	Warn about precautions	1	2

C. Prepare patient physically

		1	2
1.	Remove clothing, tape, as necessary	1	2
2.	Position patient; comfortable yet accessible	1	2

D. Prepare equipment/supplies

		1	2
1.	Set-up equipment/get supplies	1	2
2.	Prepare electrodes	1	2
3.	Check equipment operation	1	2
4.	Safety check	1	2

STEP 3. APPLICATION PARAMETERS

A. Procedures
    1. Set pulse rate (>30 pps—tetanic contraction)   1   2
    2. Set duty cycle and timer   1   2
    3. Adjust surge controls as necessary   1   2
    4. Inform patient of start/request feedback   1   2
    5. Increase until response, adjust as needed   1   2
    6. If motor point, move electrode as needed   1   2
    7. Troubleshoot discomfort   1   2
    8. Increase resistance as patient is able   1   2
B. Dosage   1   2
C. Length of application   1   2
D. Frequency of application   1   2
E. Duration of therapy   1   2

STEP 4. POSTAPPLICATION TASKS

A. Remove/replace equipment   1   2
B. Clean patient and area   1   2
C. Instructions to patient:
    1. Schedule next treatment   1   2
    2. Level of activity   1   2
    3. Self-treatment prior to next formal treatment   1   2
    4. Physiological responses following treatment   1   2
D. Record treatment and unique responses   1   2
E. Return generator cart   1   2

STEP 5. MAINTENANCE

A. Check the fuse in back of unit if not working   1   2
B. Clean equipment regularly
    1. Wash sponges or carbon-rubber electrodes   1   2
    2. Do not wash self-adhering electrodes   1   2
C. Routine maintenance
    1. Ensure wire firmly attached to electrode post   1   2
    2. Check current, assess need for new electrode   1   2

Date: _____ _____

Number correct: _____ _____

Name of Subject/Tester: _____

NMES—Twitch Contraction

Textbook Reference: Part IV, Chapter 10

Name: _____

	Application #	1	2

STEP 1. FOUNDATION

		1	2
A.	Explain NMES and basic operation	1	2
B.	Explain NMES's:		
	1. Effects	1	2
	2. Advantages	1	2
	3. Disadvantages	1	2
	4. Indications	1	2
	5. Contraindications	1	2
	6. Precautions	1	2

STEP 2. PREAPPLICATION TASKS

		1	2
A.	Ensure NMES is the proper therapy		
	1. Reevaluate and review injury	1	2
	2. Review previous application	1	2
	3. Match goals to modality	1	2
	4. Select or review electrical current	1	2
	5. Check contraindications	1	2
B.	Prepare patient psychologically		
	1. Explain procedure and expected outcomes	1	2
	2. Give brief physiology if interested	1	2
	3. Tell what to expect, what to feel	1	2
	4. Demonstrate on self if patient is apprehensive	1	2
	5. Warn about precautions	1	2
C.	Prepare patient physically		
	1. Remove clothing, tape, as necessary	1	2
	2. Position patient; comfortable yet accessible	1	2
D.	Prepare equipment/supplies		
	1. Set-up equipment/get supplies	1	2
	2. Prepare electrodes	1	2
	3. Check equipment operation	1	2
	4. Safety check	1	2

STEP 3. APPLICATION PARAMETERS

A. Procedures
    1. Set pulse rate (<10 pps for twitch contraction)   1   2
    2. Set duty cycle and timer   1   2
    3. Adjust surge controls as necessary   1   2
    4. Inform patient of start/request feedback   1   2
    5. Increase until response, adjust as needed   1   2
    6. If motor point, move electrode as needed   1   2
    7. Troubleshoot discomfort   1   2
    8. Increase resistance as patient is able   1   2
B. Dosage   1   2
C. Length of application   1   2
D. Frequency of application   1   2
E. Duration of therapy   1   2

STEP 4. POSTAPPLICATION TASKS

A. Remove/replace equipment   1   2
B. Clean patient and area   1   2
C. Instructions to patient:
    1. Schedule next treatment   1   2
    2. Level of activity   1   2
    3. Self-treatment prior to next formal treatment   1   2
    4. Physiological responses following treatment   1   2
D. Record treatment and unique responses   1   2
E. Return generator cart   1   2

STEP 5. MAINTENANCE

A. Check the fuse in back of unit if not working   1   2
B. Clean equipment regularly
    1. Wash sponges or carbon-rubber electrodes   1   2
    2. Do not wash self-adhering electrodes   1   2
C. Routine maintenance
    1. Ensure wire firmly attached to electrode post   1   2
    2. Check current, assess need for new electrode   1   2

Date: _____ _____

Number correct: _____ _____

Name of Subject/Tester: _____

Whirlpool

Textbook Reference: Part V, Ch. 12

Name: _____

STEP 1. FOUNDATION

A.	Explain whirlpool and basic operation	1	2
B.	Explain the whirlpool's:		
	1. Effects	1	2
	2. Advantages	1	2
	3. Disadvantages	1	2
	4. Indications	1	2
	5. Contraindications	1	2
	6. Precautions	1	2

STEP 2. PREAPPLICATION TASKS

A.	Ensure whirlpool is the proper therapy		
	1. Reevaluate and review injury	1	2
	2. Review previous application	1	2
	3. Match goals to modality	1	2
	4. Check contraindications	1	2
B.	Prepare equipment/supplies		
	1. Set-up equipment (drain, temperature)	1	2
	2. Check whirlpool electrical operation	1	2
	3. Add disinfectant/antacid	1	2
	4. Safety check	1	2
C.	Prepare patient psychologically		
	1. Explain procedure and expected outcomes	1	2
	2. Give brief physiology if interested	1	2
	3. Tell what to expect, what to feel	1	2
	4. Check for, and warn about, precautions	1	2
D.	Prepare patient physically		
	1. Remove clothing, tape, as necessary	1	2
	2. Position patient; comfortable yet accessible	1	2

STEP 3. APPLICATION PARAMETERS

A. Procedures

1.	Turn on turbine before patient gets in water	1	2
2.	Help patient in if needed	1	2
3.	Adjust turbine height and readjust patient	1	2
4.	Adjust direction of water flow	1	2
5.	Do not leave patient unattended	1	2
6.	Turn off turbine before patient gets out	1	2

B.	Dosage	1	2
C.	Length of application	1	2
D.	Frequency of application	1	2
E.	Duration of therapy	1	2

STEP 4. POSTAPPLICATION TASKS

A. Instructions to patient

1.	Schedule next treatment	1	2
2.	Instruct about level of activity	1	2
3.	Rehydrate after warm, full-body whirlpool	1	2

B.	Record treatment and unique responses	1	2

C. Whirlpool and area cleanup

1.	Wipe water off benches and clean floor	1	2
2.	Drain tank at end of day	1	2
3.	Clean and disinfect whirlpool daily	1	2

STEP 5. MAINTENANCE

A.	Keep equipment clean and polished	1	2
B.	Check electrical cord for fraying	1	2

Date: _____ _____

Number correct: _____ _____

Name of Subject/Tester: _____

Hot Pack

Textbook Reference: Part V, Chapter 12

Name: _____

STEP 1. FOUNDATION

A.	Explain the hot pack and basic operation	1	2
B.	Explain the hot pack's:		
	1. Effects	1	2
	2. Advantages	1	2
	3. Disadvantages	1	2
	4. Indications	1	2
	5. Contraindications	1	2
	6. Precautions	1	2

STEP 2. PREAPPLICATION TASKS

A.	Ensure hot packs are the proper therapy		
	1. Reevaluate and review injury	1	2
	2. Review previous application	1	2
	3. Match goals to modality	1	2
	4. Check contraindications	1	2
B.	Prepare patient psychologically		
	1. Explain procedure and expected outcomes	1	2
	2. Give brief physiology if interested	1	2
	3. Tell what to expect, what to feel	1	2
	4. Check for, and warn about, precautions	1	2
C.	Prepare patient physically		
	1. Let patient decide whether to remove clothing	1	2
	2. Position patient; comfortable yet accessible	1	2
D.	Prepare equipment/supplies		
	1. Ensure heating unit is at proper temperature	1	2
	2. Have adequate toweling available	1	2
	3. Hours before, presoak and preheat packs	1	2
	4. Just before, remove heating pack from unit	1	2
	5. Prepare pack on table, not on patient	1	2

STEP 3. APPLICATION PARAMETERS

A. Procedures
    1. Place prepared pack on patient   1   2
    2. Place another towel over pack   1   2
    3. Check patient every 4–5 minutes   1   2
B. Dosage   1   2
C. Length of application   1   2
D. Frequency of application   1   2
E. Duration of therapy   1   2

STEP 4. POSTAPPLICATION TASKS

A. Instructions to patient:
    1. Schedule next treatment   1   2
    2. Instruct about level of activity   1   2
B. Record treatment and unique responses   1   2
C. Replace and cleanup equipment
    1. Return packs to heating unit immediately   1   2
    2. Return towels to drying rack or laundry   1   2

STEP 5. MAINTENANCE

A. Clean heating unit at least once a month   1   2
B. Routine maintenance
    1. Keep water level in heating unit above packs   1   2
    2. Do not allow packs to dry out   1   2
    3. Check thermostat yearly for proper operation   1   2
C. Watch packs for loss of gel as result of wear   1   2

Date: _____ _____

Number correct: _____ _____

Name of Subject/Tester: _____

Paraffin Bath

Textbook Reference: Part V, Chapter 12

Name: _____

STEP 1. FOUNDATION

A.	Explain paraffin bath and basic operation	1	2
B.	Explain the paraffin bath's:		
	1. Effects	1	2
	2. Advantages	1	2
	3. Disadvantages	1	2
	4. Indications	1	2
	5. Contraindications	1	2
	6. Precautions	1	2

STEP 2. PREAPPLICATION TASKS

A.	Ensure paraffin bath is the proper therapy		
	1. Reevaluate and review injury	1	2
	2. Review previous application	1	2
	3. Match goals to modality	1	2
	4. Check contraindications	1	2
B.	Prepare patient psychologically		
	1. Explain procedure and expected outcomes	1	2
	2. Give brief physiology if interested	1	2
	3. Tell what to expect, what to feel	1	2
	4. Check for, and warn about, precautions	1	2
C.	Prepare patient physically		
	1. Remove all clothing, jewelry, tape from area.	1	2
	2. Ensure skin is clean/dry	1	2
	3. Cover small scratches	1	2
	4. Place a towel over clothing	1	2
D.	Prepare equipment/supplies		
	1. Hours before, prepare paraffin	1	2
	2. Check/adjust temperature as needed	1	2
	3. Immediately before, recheck temperature	1	2

STEP 3. APPLICATION PARAMETERS

A. Procedures

    1. Dip body part in paraffin and remove   1   2

    2. Allow paraffin to cool   1   2

    3. Repeat for 7 to 12 total layers   1   2

    4. Cover area with cellophane or plastic bag and then a towel   1   2

B. Dosage   1   2

C. Length of application   1   2

D. Frequency of application   1   2

E. Duration of therapy   1   2

STEP 4. POSTAPPLICATION TASKS

A. Instructions to patient:

    1. Schedule next treatment   1   2

    2. Instruct about level of activity   1   2

B. Record treatment and unique responses   1   2

C. Remove equipment/clean patient

    1. Peel paraffin from body; discard/put in bath   1   2

STEP 5. MAINTENANCE

A. Check paraffin bath for foreign material/remove   1   2

B. Replace paraffin as it is used   1   2

Date: _____ _____

Number correct: _____ _____

Name of Subject/Tester: _____

Cryokinetics

Textbook Reference: Part V, Chapter 14

Name: _____

STEP 1. FOUNDATION

A. Explain cryokinetics and basic application   1   2
B. Explain cryokinetics':
    1. Effects   1   2
    2. Advantages   1   2
    3. Disadvantages   1   2
    4. Indications   1   2
    5. Contraindications   1   2
    6. Precautions   1   2

STEP 2. PREAPPLICATION TASKS

A. Ensure cryokinetics is the proper therapy
    1. Reevaluate and review injury   1   2
    2. Review previous application   1   2
    3. Match goals to modality   1   2
    4. Check contraindications   1   2
B. Prepare patient psychologically
    1. Explain procedure and expected outcomes   1   2
    2. Give brief physiology if interested   1   2
    3. Tell what to expect, what to feel   1   2
C. Prepare patient physically
    1. Remove necessary clothing   1   2
    2. Position patient; comfortable yet accessible   1   2
D. Prepare equipment/supplies
    1. Have container, ice/popsicle available   1   2
    2. Have toe cap if possible (not necessary)   1   2
    3. Have towel to clean melting ice   1   2

STEP 3. APPLICATION PARAMETERS

A. Procedures
    1. Numb body part by applying ice   1   2
    2. Exercise area as long as it is numb   1   2
    3. Reapply ice until numb again   1   2
    4. Exercise injured area   1   2
    5. Principles: active, progressive, pain-free   1   2
B. Dosage   1   2
C. Length of application   1   2
D. Frequency of application   1   2
E. Duration of therapy   1   2

STEP 4. POSTAPPLICATION TASKS

A.   Instructions to patient:
    1.   Instruct to use same supportive devices   1   2
    2.   Instruct about level of activity   1   2
    3.   Explain pain may return, use ice pack   1   2
    4.   Schedule next treatment   1   2
B.   Record treatment and unique responses   1   2
C.   Clean area
    1.   Put away ice container, towel, etc.   1   2
    2.   Wipe water from floor   1   2

STEP 5. MAINTENANCE

A.   Replace slush container when cracked   1   2
B.   Sew sides of toe caps if they rip   1   2

Date: _____ _____

Number correct: _____ _____

Name of Subject/Tester: _____

Cryostretch

Textbook Reference: Part V, Chapter 14

Name: _____

STEP 1. FOUNDATION

A.	Explain cryostretch and basic application	1	2
B.	Explain cryostretch's:		
	1. Effects	1	2
	2. Advantages	1	2
	3. Disadvantages	1	2
	4. Indications	1	2
	5. Contraindications	1	2
	6. Precautions	1	2

STEP 2. PREAPPLICATION TASKS

A.	Ensure cryostretch is the proper therapy		
	1. Reevaluate and review injury	1	2
	2. Review previous application	1	2
	3. Match goals to modality	1	2
	4. Check contraindications	1	2
B.	Prepare patient psychologically		
	1. Explain procedure and expected outcomes	1	2
	2. Give brief physiology if interested	1	2
	3. Tell what to expect, what to feel	1	2
C.	Prepare patient physically		
	1. Remove necessary clothing	1	2
	2. Position patient; comfortable yet accessible	1	2
D.	Prepare equipment/supplies		
	1. Have container, ice/popsicle available	1	2
	2. Have toe cap if possible (not necessary)	1	2
	3. Have towel to clean melting ice	1	2

STEP 3. APPLICATION PARAMETERS

A.	Procedures		
	1. Applying ice to body part until numb	1	2
	2. Stretch muscles as long as they are numb	1	2
	3. Reapply ice until numb again	1	2
	4. Exercise injured area	1	2
	5. Passive stretching and static contraction	1	2
B.	Dosage	1	2
C.	Length of application	1	2
D.	Frequency of application	1	2
E.	Duration of therapy	1	2

STEP 4. POSTAPPLICATION TASKS

A. Instructions to patient:
    1. Instruct to use same supportive devices   1   2
    2. Instruct about level of activity   1   2
    3. Explain pain may return, use ice pack   1   2
    4. Schedule next treatment   1   2
B. Record treatment and unique responses   1   2
C. Clean area
    1. Put away ice container, towel, etc.   1   2
    2. Wipe water from floor   1   2

STEP 5. MAINTENANCE

None

Date: _____   _____

Number correct: _____   _____

Name of Subject/Tester: _____

Lymph Edema Pump

Textbook Reference: Part V, Chapter 14

Name: _____

STEP 1. FOUNDATION

A.	Explain lymph edema pump and basic operation	1	2
B.	Explain the lymph edema pump's:		
	1. Effects	1	2
	2. Advantages	1	2
	3. Disadvantages	1	2
	4. Indications	1	2
	5. Contraindications	1	2
	6. Precautions	1	2
	7. Alternatives	1	2

STEP 2. PREAPPLICATION TASKS

A.	Ensure lymph edema pump is the proper therapy		
	1. Reevaluate and review injury	1	2
	2. Review previous application	1	2
	3. Match goals to modality	1	2
	4. Check contraindications	1	2
B.	Prepare patient psychologically		
	1. Explain procedure and expected outcomes	1	2
	2. Give brief physiology if interested	1	2
	3. Tell what to expect, what to feel	1	2
C.	Prepare patient physically		
	1. Remove necessary clothing	1	2
	2. Position patient; comfortable yet accessible	1	2
D.	Prepare equipment/supplies		
	1. Have container, ice/popsicle available	1	2
	2. Have toe cap if possible (not necessary)	1	2
	3. Have towel to clean melting ice	1	2

STEP 3. APPLICATION PARAMETERS

A. Procedures
    1. Applying sleeve to extremity, tighten   1   2
    2. Attach sleeve tube to pump   1   2
    3. If using water device, fill with ice and water   1   2
    4. Select on/off times   1   2
    5. Turn on device   1   2
B. Dosage   1   2
C. Length of application   1   2
D. Frequency of application   1   2
E. Duration of therapy   1   2

STEP 4. POSTAPPLICATION TASKS

A. Instructions to patient:
    1. Schedule next treatment   1   2
    2. Instruct about level of activity   1   2
B. Record treatment and unique responses   1   2
C. Clean area
    1. Remove equipment   1   2
    2. Clean inside of cuff or boot with disinfectant   1   2

STEP 5. MAINTENANCE

A. Check hoses, valves, boots, sleeves for leaks   1   2

Date: _____ _____

Number correct: _____ _____

Name of Subject/Tester: _____

		ACTIVITY
Ultrasound		**29**

Textbook Reference: Part V, Chapter 15

Name: _____

STEP 1. FOUNDATION

A.	Explain ultrasound and basic operation	1	2
B.	Explain ultrasound's:		
	1. Effects	1	2
	2. Advantages	1	2
	3. Disadvantages	1	2
	4. Indications	1	2
	5. Contraindications	1	2
	6. Precautions	1	2

STEP 2. PREAPPLICATION TASKS

A.	Ensure ultrasound is the proper therapy		
	1. Reevaluate and review injury	1	2
	2. Review previous application	1	2
	3. Match goals to modality	1	2
	4. Check contraindications	1	2
B.	Prepare equipment/supplies		
	1. Ensure soundhead is clean	1	2
	2. Have enough coupling medium for treatment	1	2
C.	Prepare patient psychologically		
	1. Explain procedure and expected outcomes	1	2
	2. Give brief physiology if interested	1	2
	3. Tell what to expect, what to feel	1	2
	4. Demonstrate on self if patient is apprehensive	1	2
	5. Warn about precautions	1	2
D.	Prepare patient physically		
	1. Remove metal, jewelry from area	1	2
	2. Inspect area for rashes, open wounds	1	2
	3. Position patient; comfortable yet accessible	1	2

STEP 3. APPLICATION PARAMETERS

A.	Procedures		
	1. Obtain appropriate soundhead size	1	2
	2. Apply coupling medium to area	1	2
	3. Begin moving soundhead and turn on	1	2
B.	Dosage	1	2
C.	Length of application	1	2
D.	Frequency of application	1	2
E.	Duration of therapy	1	2

STEP 4. POSTAPPLICATION TASKS

A. Remove equipment/clean patient
    1. Remove soundhead and clean   1   2
    2. Wipe ultrasound gel off patient   1   2
B. Instructions to patient:
    1. Schedule next treatment   1   2
    2. Instruct about level of activity   1   2
    3. Explain what patient may feel after treatment   1   2
C. Record treatment and unique responses   1   2
D. Replace equipment
    1. Towels   1   2
    2. Coupling medium   1   2

STEP 5. MAINTENANCE

A. Clean equipment regularly   1   2
B. Calibrate every six months if used daily   1   2

Date: _____ _____

Number correct: _____ _____

Name of Subject/Tester: _____

Pulsed Shortwave Diathermy (PSWD)

Textbook Reference: Part V, Chapter 16

Name: _____

STEP 1. FOUNDATION

A.	Explain PSWD and basic operation	1	2
B.	Explain PSWD's:		
	1. Effects	1	2
	2. Advantages	1	2
	3. Disadvantages	1	2
	4. Indications	1	2
	5. Contraindications	1	2
	6. Precautions	1	2

STEP 2. PREAPPLICATION TASKS

A.	Ensure PSWD is the proper therapy		
	1. Reevaluate and review injury	1	2
	2. Review previous application	1	2
	3. Match goals to modality	1	2
B.	Prepare equipment/supplies		
	1. Ensure drum/applicator is clean and dry	1	2
C.	Prepare patient psychologically		
	1. Explain procedure and expected outcomes	1	2
	2. Give brief physiology if interested	1	2
	3. Tell what to expect, what to feel	1	2
	4. Demonstrate on self if patient is apprehensive	1	2
	5. Warn about precautions	1	2
D.	Prepare patient physically		
	1. Remove metal, jewelry, and moisture from area	1	2
	2. Remove synthetic fabrics	1	2
	3. Position patient; comfortable yet accessible	1	2
	4. Inspect area for rashes, open wounds	1	2

STEP 3. APPLICATION PARAMETERS

A.	Procedures		
	1. Place drum/applicator on area	1	2
	2. Turn device on	1	2
B.	Dosage	1	2
C.	Length of application	1	2
D.	Frequency of application	1	2
E.	Duration of therapy	1	2

STEP 4. POSTAPPLICATION TASKS

A. Equipment removal
    1. As timer sounds, ensure all knobs are at zero   1   2
B. Instructions to patient:
    1. Schedule next treatment   1   2
    2. Instruct about level of activity   1   2
    3. Explain what patient may feel after treatment   1   2
C. Record treatment and unique responses   1   2
D. Replace equipment
    1. Clean table, removing sweat or moisture   1   2
    2. Replace used towels   1   2

STEP 5. MAINTENANCE

A. Clean equipment regularly   1   2
B. Ensure all cables/connections work   1   2

Date: _____ _____

Number correct: _____ _____

Name of Subject/Tester: _____

Massage

Textbook Reference: Part VI, Chapter 17

Name: _____

STEP 1. FOUNDATION

A. Explain massage and basic application	1	2
B. Explain massage's:		
1. Effects	1	2
2. Advantages	1	2
3. Disadvantages	1	2
4. Indications	1	2
5. Contraindications	1	2
6. Precautions	1	2

STEP 2. PREAPPLICATION TASKS

A. Ensure massage is the proper therapy		
1. (Re)evaluate and review previous application	1	2
2. Establish goals	1	2
3. Match goals to modality	1	2
4. Check contraindications	1	2
B. Prepare patient psychologically		
1. Explain benefits	1	2
2. Tell what to expect; reassure modesty	1	2
C. Prepare patient physically		
1. Ensure suitable environment (warm, relaxed)	1	2
2. Position patient; comfortable yet accessible	1	2
3. Ensure patient is properly draped	1	2
D. Prepare equipment/supplies		
1. Determine type of massage, what order	1	2
2. Determine whether to use lubricants	1	2

STEP 3. APPLICATION PARAMETERS

A. Procedures for "typical" sports massage application		
1. Light effleurage	1	2
2. Deep effleurage	1	2
3. Petrissage	1	2
4. Optional friction/percussion	1	2
5. Deep petrissage	1	2
6. Light effleurage	1	2
B. Dosage	1	2
C. Length of application	1	2
D. Frequency of application	1	2
E. Duration of therapy	1	2

STEP 4. POSTAPPLICATION TASKS

A. Equipment removal
    1. Remove remaining massage lubricant   1   2
B. Instructions to patient:
    1. Schedule next treatment   1   2
    2. Instruct about level of activity   1   2
C. Record treatment and unique responses   1   2
D. Replace soiled towels/sheets with clean ones   1   2

STEP 5. MAINTENANCE

A. Keep hands free of calluses   1   2
B. Ensure massage tables are in working order   1   2
C. Ensure plenty of massage lubricant for future   1   2

Date: _____ _____

Number correct: _____ _____

Name of Subject/Tester: _____

Cervical Traction	ACTIVITY **32**

Textbook Reference: Book Part VI, Chapter 18

Name: _____

STEP 1. FOUNDATION

A. Explain cervical traction and basic application	1 2
B. Explain cervical traction's:	
1. Effects	1 2
2. Advantages	1 2
3. Disadvantages	1 2
4. Indications	1 2
5. Contraindications	1 2
6. Precautions	1 2

STEP 2. PREAPPLICATION TASKS

A. Ensure traction is the proper therapy	
1. (Re)evaluate and review previous application	1 2
2. Establish goals	1 2
3. Match goals to modality	1 2
4. Check contraindications	1 2
B. Prepare patient psychologically	
1. Explain pulling sensation	1 2
2. Tell to expect relieved pressure and pain	1 2
C. Prepare patient physically	
1. Remove clothing, jewelry, bandages, etc.	1 2
2. Secure head harness to patient	1 2
3. Ensure patient is properly positioned	1 2
D. Prepare mechanical equipment, if using	
1. See user manual for specific setups	1 2
2. Ensure the machine is operating properly	1 2
3. Ensure displayed traction is correct	1 2
4. Ensure that duty cycle is operating correctly	1 2

STEP 3. APPLICATION PARAMETERS

A. Procedures for manual/mechanical cervical traction	
1. Support head	1 2
2. Clinician/machine applies intermittent force	1 2
B. Dosage	1 2
C. Length of application	1 2
D. Frequency of application	1 2
E. Duration of therapy	1 2

STEP 4. POSTAPPLICATION TASKS

A. Equipment removal
    1.   Remove harnesses or belts   1   2
    2.   Turn off machine   1   2
B. Instructions to patient:
    1.   Schedule next treatment   1   2
    2.   Instruct about level of activity   1   2
    3.   Instruct how patient should feel after   1   2
C. Record treatment and unique responses   1   2
D. Clean off table (if used)   1   2

STEP 5. MAINTENANCE

A. Periodically check belts, harnesses, etc.   1   2

Date: _____ _____

Number correct: _____ _____

Name of Subject/Tester: _____

Lumbar Traction

Textbook Reference: Book Part VI, Chapter 18

Name: _____

STEP 1. FOUNDATION

A.	Explain lumbar traction and basic application	1	2
B.	Explain lumbar traction's:		
	1. Effects	1	2
	2. Advantages	1	2
	3. Disadvantages	1	2
	4. Indications	1	2
	5. Contraindications	1	2
	6. Precautions	1	2

STEP 2. PREAPPLICATION TASKS

A.	Ensure traction is the proper therapy		
	1. (Re)evaluate and review previous application	1	2
	2. Establish goals	1	2
	3. Match goals to modality	1	2
	4. Check contraindications	1	2
B.	Prepare patient psychologically		
	1. Explain pulling sensation	1	2
	2. Tell to expect relieved pressure and pain	1	2
C.	Prepare patient physically		
	1. Remove clothing, jewelry, bandages, etc.	1	2
	2. Secure chest and pelvic harness to patient	1	2
	3. Ensure patient is properly positioned	1	2
D.	Prepare mechanical equipment, if using		
	1. See user manual for specific setups	1	2
	2. Ensure the machine is operating properly	1	2
	3. Ensure displayed traction is correct	1	2
	4. Ensure that duty cycle is operating correctly	1	2

STEP 3. APPLICATION PARAMETERS

A.	Procedures for manual lumbar traction		
	1. Clinician/machine applies intermittent force	1	2
	2. Steady pull until noticeable distraction felt	1	2
B.	Dosage	1	2
C.	Length of application	1	2
D.	Frequency of application	1	2
E.	Duration of therapy	1	2

STEP 4. POSTAPPLICATION TASKS

A.   Equipment removal
    1.   Remove harnesses or belts   1   2
    2.   Turn off machine   1   2
B.   Instructions to patient:
    1.   Schedule next treatment   1   2
    2.   Instruct about level of activity   1   2
    3.   Instruct how patient should feel after   1   2
C.   Record treatment and unique responses   1   2
D.   Clean off table (if used)   1   2

STEP 5. MAINTENANCE

A.   Periodically check belts, harnesses, etc.   1   2

Date: _____ _____

Number correct: _____ _____

Name of Subject/Tester: _____

Light Therapy	ACTIVITY
	34

Textbook Reference: Part VI, Chapter 19

Name: _____

STEP 1. FOUNDATION

A.	Explain light therapy and basic operation	1	2
B.	Explain light therapy's:		
	1. Effects	1	2
	2. Advantages	1	2
	3. Disadvantages	1	2
	4. Indications	1	2
	5. Contraindications	1	2
	6. Precautions	1	2

STEP 2. PREAPPLICATION TASKS

A.	Ensure light therapy is the proper therapy	1	2
B.	Prepare patient psychologically		
	1. Explain that no sensation should be felt	1	2
C.	Prepare patient physically		
	1. Remove clothing, jewelry, bandages, etc.	1	2
	2. Clean and dry skin of treatment	1	2
D.	Equipment preparation		
	1. Check manual for average power output	1	2
	2. Calculate treatment time	1	2
	3. Ensure machine is operating properly	1	2
	4. Ensure displayed time is correct	1	2
	5. Ensure pulse rate is set properly, if applicable	1	2

STEP 3. APPLICATION PARAMETERS

A.	Procedures		
	1. Turn on machine/adjust output parameters	1	2
	2. Wear safety goggles, if using laser	1	2
	3. Apply directly to skin except open wound	1	2
	4. For large areas, use cluster, grid, or scanning	1	2
B.	Dosage	1	2
C.	Length of application	1	2
D.	Frequency of application	1	2
E.	Duration of therapy	1	2

STEP 4. POSTAPPLICATION TASKS

A.	Equipment removal/patient cleanup	1	2
B.	Instructions to patient:		
	1. Schedule next treatment	1	2
	2. Instruct about level of activity	1	2
	3. Instruct how patient should feel after	1	2
C.	Record treatment and unique responses	1	2
D.	Clean off table (if used)	1	2
E.	Replace equipment/cleanup area	1	2

STEP 5. MAINTENANCE

A.	Regularly clean equipment	1	2
B.	Perform routine maintenance	1	2
C.	Perform simple repairs	1	2

Date: _____ _____

Number correct: _____ _____

Name of Subject/Tester: _____